Try It Now! GREEN SMOOTHIES

by Howard Mills

Table of Contents

8. Organic Orange & Spinach Green Smoothie

9. Banana Ginger & Orange Green Spinach Smoothie

10. Blueberry Mint Kiwi Green Smoothie

11. Sweet Honeydew Melon & Mint Green Smoothie

12. Pomegranate Banana Citrus Green Spinach Smoothie

13. Pineapple Banana Green Kale Smoothie

14. Mango Jalapeno Pepper Green Smoothie

15. Mojito Mint Green Smoothie

1. Introduction

Hello and welcome to the healthy eating lifestyle. Thank you for downloading my book. This amazing book contains a compiled list of **20 High Quality Green Smoothie** recipes that will make your taste buds dance. These Green Smoothie recipes will hold your hand and guide you down the path of healthy living. **Hope you All enjoy!**

2. Hemp Seed Banana Mango Green Smoothie Bowls

Hemp Seed Banana Mango Green Smoothie Bowls

Servings 2

Ingredients:

- 2 bananas

- 3 large handfuls baby kale or spinach

- 1 handful of micro-greens or sprouts

- 1 mango, peeled + cubed

- 3 tablespoons hemp seeds

- ½ cup unsweetened almond milk {or preferred milk}

- 2 -3 ice cubes

Directions:

1. Blend all of the ingredients until smooth.
2. Divide the smoothie into two bowls.
3. Top with additional garnishes.

Garnish options:

- fresh mango slices, or other seasonal fruit
- hemp seeds
- chia seeds
- sprouts
- micro-greens
- shredded coconut
- honey
- buckwheat groats
- goji berries

3. Protein Warrior Green Smoothie

Protein Warrior Green Smoothie

Servings 1-2

- 1/2 cup fresh red grapefruit juice*

- 1 cup kale or baby spinach**

- 1 large sweet apple, cored and roughly chopped

- 1 cup chopped cucumber

- 1 medium/large stalk celery, chopped (about 3/4 cup)

- 3 to 4 tablespoons hemp hearts, to taste

- 1/3 cup frozen mango

- 2 tablespoons packed fresh mint leaves

- 1 1/2 teaspoons virgin coconut oil (optional)

- 4 ice cubes, or as needed

Directions:

1. Juice a red grapefruit and add 1/2 cup grapefruit juice to the blender.

2. Now add the kale (or spinach), apple, cucumber, celery, hemp, mango, mint, coconut oil (if using), and ice. Blend on high until super smooth. (If using a Vita mix, use the tamper stick to push it down until it blends). You can add a bit of water if necessary to get it blending.

3. Pour into a glass.

4. Mango Vegan Green Smoothie

Mango Vegan Green Smoothie

Servings 1-2

Ingredients:

- 1 cup fresh washed spinach leaves, packed
- 1 cup fresh or frozen mango cubes
- 1/2 medium banana
- 3/4 cup light canned coconut
- 1/2 cup orange juice
- 1/2 cup ice cubes

Directions:

1. Place all ingredients in a blender and puree until smooth. Pour into glasses, add toppings if desired, and serve with a straw.

5. Leprechaun Mint Green Smoothie

Leprechaun Mint Green Smoothie

Servings 1

Ingredients:

- ½ average avocado

- ¼ cup coconut milk, organic (or full-fat cream)

- ¼ cup fresh baby spinach

- fresh mint or mint extract to taste

- ¼ cup vanilla or plain whey protein or egg white protein powder

- 2 tbsp pistachio nuts (unsalted)

- 1 vanilla bean or ½ - 1 tsp vanilla extract

- 3-6 drops liquid Stevia

- ½ cup water

- ice cubes (if needed)

Directions:

1. Wash the mint and spinach, halve and peel the avocado and blend until smooth with the rest of the ingredients.

6. Tropical Fruit Green Spinach Smoothie

Tropical Fruit Green Spinach Smoothie

Servings 1-2

Ingredients:

- 1 to 2 cups frozen spinach

- 1 cup frozen pineapple chunks

- 1 cup frozen mango chunks

- 1 medium ripe banana, peeled

- 1 cup strawberries, blueberries, raspberries, or a favorite berry, optional

- 1 cup milk (cow's, almond, soy, coconut, kefir, horchata)

- 1 teaspoon + vanilla extract

- sweetener, to taste (sugar, agave, stevia, honey, maple syrup, Medjool dates).

Directions:

1. All ingredients and amounts are to taste. Use seasonal fruits or vary the quantities of fruits, to taste.

2. Place all ingredients in the canister of a Vita-Mix or blender and blend until smooth and creamy. Serve immediately. Freeze extra portions.

7. Peanut Butter Yogurt Green Smoothie

Peanut Butter Yogurt Green Smoothie

Servings 1-2

Ingredients:

- 1 ripe banana
- 1 1/2 cups fresh spinach
- 1 cup frozen blueberries
- 1/4 cup yogurt
- splash of milk
- 1/2 tablespoon creamy peanut butter
- 1 tablespoon chia seeds

Directions:

1. Blend all ingredients in blender until smooth. Add more blueberries if you want your smoothie a little thicker. Once smooth, add chia seeds and pulse several times. Serve.

8. Organic Orange & Spinach Green Smoothie

Organic Orange & Spinach Green Smoothie

Servings 1

Ingredients:

- 1 navel orange, peeled

- 1/2 banana, peeled

- 1 cup tightly packed organic spinach

- 1/4 cup coconut water, adjusted as desired

- 1 tablespoon hemp seeds, optional

- Ice

Directions:

1. Add all ingredients to a blender with a few ice cubes and blend on high to combine.

2. Add more coconut water as desired to reach desired consistency for smoothie.

3. Pour into a glass and serve.

9. Banana Ginger & Orange Green Spinach Smoothie

Banana Ginger & Orange Green Spinach Smoothie

Servings 2

Ingredients:

- 1 1/2 cups filtered water
- 4 generous handfuls fresh spinach
- 4 romaine leaves (optional)
- 2 navel oranges
- 2 ripe bananas
- 1"-2" knob of fresh ginger
- 1 cucumber (optional) peel if not organic

Directions:

1. Rinse and prep veggies.

2. Mix everything in the blender and blend until smooth.

3. Pour into a glass and serve.

10. Blueberry Mint Kiwi Green Smoothie

Blueberry Mint Kiwi Green Smoothie

Servings 1

Ingredients:

- 2 cups spinach

- 2 cups blueberry

- 1 kiwi

- 3-4 large mint leaves

- 1 cup coconut water

- 1 cup ice

Directions:

1. Put all ingredients in a blender and mix it up then serve.

11. Sweet Honeydew Melon & Mint Green Smoothie

Sweet Honeydew Melon & Mint Green Smoothie

Servings 4

Ingredients:

- 1/2 honeydew melon, cut into chunks (about 4 cups, or 1 1/2 lbs)

- 1/2 cup light coconut milk

- 1-2 leaves fresh mint

- 1/2-1 tsp. fresh lime juice (or to taste)

- 1 cup ice

- Drizzle of honey or coconut nectar, to taste

Directions:

1. Cut your melon in half, remove the seeds, and slice away the outer rind. Cut the melon into chunks, and add to your blender along with the coconut milk, mint, lime, and ice. Blend until smooth. Taste, and adjust sweetness with honey or coconut nectar. Serve with a garnish of mint, or fresh melon slices.

12. Pomegranate Banana Citrus Green Spinach Smoothie

Pomegranate Banana Citrus Green Spinach Smoothie

Servings 1-2

Ingredients:

- 2 cups spinach, fresh

- 1 cup water

- 2 oranges, peeled

- 1 cup pomegranate seeds

- 2 bananas

- Ice

Directions:

1. Blend spinach and water until smooth.

2. Next add the fruits and blend again.

3. serve.

13. Pineapple Banana Green Kale Smoothie

Pineapple Banana Green Kale Smoothie

Servings 2

Ingredients:

- ½ cup coconut milk

- 2 cups stemmed and chopped kale

- 1½ cups chopped pineapple (about ¼ medium pineapple)

- 1 ripe banana, chopped

Directions:

1. Combine the coconut milk, ½ cup water, the kale, pineapple, and banana in a blender and puree until smooth. Then Serve.

14. Mango Jalapeno Pepper Green Smoothie

Mango Jalapeno Pepper Green Smoothie

Servings 2

Ingredients:

- 2 bananas, broken into chunks

- 2 cups baby spinach

- 1 cup frozen mango chunks

- 1/2 teaspoon chopped jalapeno pepper, or to taste

- 1 cup water, or as desired

Directions:

1. Layer banana, spinach, mango, and jalapeno pepper in a blender; add water and blend until smooth, adding more water for a thinner smoothie. Serve.

15. Mojito Mint Green Smoothie

Mojito Mint Green Smoothie

Servings 2

Ingredients:

- 1 cup coconut water or water
- 1 teaspoon finely grated lime zest 3 limes, peeled and quartered
- 1 cup torn-up curly green kale leaves (1 or 2 large leaves with stalk removed)
- ½ cup firmly packed mint
- 2 cups frozen pineapple
- 5 drops alcohol-free liquid stevia, plus more to taste
- 1 teaspoon wheatgrass powder

- 1 teaspoon minced ginger

- 1 teaspoon coconut oil

Directions:

1. Throw all of the ingredients into your blender and blast on high for 30 to 60 seconds, until smooth and creamy. Serve.

16. Pineapple Kale Mojito Green Smoothie

Pineapple Kale Mojito Green Smoothie

Servings 2

Ingredients:

- 2 cups kale
- 2 cups coconut water
- 3 cups pineapple
- ¼ cup fresh mint leaves
- Juice of 1 lime

Directions:

1. Blend kale and coconut water until smooth.

2. Add remaining ingredients, and blend until smooth. Serve.

*Use frozen fruit or ice to make smoothie cold.

17. Apple Banana Yogurt Green Smoothie

Apple Banana Yogurt Green Smoothie

Servings 1

Ingredients:

- 1 small or half of a large apple, peeled and cored

- 1 frozen banana

- 1/3 cup vanilla almond milk

- 1/3 cup Greek yogurt (vanilla or plain)

- 1 cup or generous handful of baby spinach

- 2 tablespoons of raw almonds

- 2 teaspoons of honey

Directions:

1. Place all of the ingredients in your blender. Blend until smooth. Serve.

18. Spicy Avocado Green Smoothie

Spicy Avocado Green Smoothie

Servings 1-2

Ingredients:

- 1 ½ cup dairy free milk
- 1 cup mixed greens
- ¼ cup berries, fresh or frozen
- ½ avocado
- 1 tablespoon peeled ginger root
- 1 tablespoon raw honey or stevia (optional)
- 1 tablespoon ground flax seeds
- Dash cayenne pepper
- Juice from 1 lemon

Directions:

Put all ingredients in blender and mix until smooth. Serve.

19. Spicy Chia Seed Green Smoothie

Spicy Chia Seed Green Smoothie

Servings 1-2

Ingredients:

- 1 cup water

- 1/2 medium avocado

- 1 cup baby spinach (or kale)

- 1/2 cup fresh or frozen blueberries

- 1 tablespoon chia seeds or chia seed gel

- 1/2 tablespoon coconut oil

- 1/4 teaspoon chili powder

- 1/2 tablespoon honey

Directions:

1. Place all of the ingredients into your high-speed blender and blend for around 30-45 seconds or until nice and smooth. Serve.

20. Cashew Chai Spice Green Smoothie

Cashew Chai Spice Green Smoothie

Servings 2

Ingredients:

- 3 tablespoons cashews

- 2 tablespoons hemp seeds

- 2 Medjool dates

- 2 tablespoons cacao nibs

- 1 teaspoon wheatgrass

- 1 cup spinach

- 1 teaspoon cinnamon

- 1 teaspoon ground cardamom

- 1 teaspoon ground ginger

- ¼ teaspoon ground cloves

- 1 cup coconut water

- 1 cup unsweetened almond milk

- 1 frozen banana

- 1 cup ice

Directions:

1. Combine all ingredients into a large, high-powered blender and blend until smooth and creamy.

2. Then serve.

21. Pear Yogurt Green Spinach Smoothie

Pear Yogurt Green Spinach Smoothie

Servings 2

Ingredients:

- 1 cup unsweetened almond milk or milk of choice
- 1 cup spinach
- 1 heaping cup diced frozen pears
- 1/2 cup plain non-fat Greek yogurt
- 1 tablespoon almond butter
- Honey to taste
- 1/2 teaspoon fresh grated ginger
- 1/2 teaspoon vanilla extract

Directions:

1. Place all of the ingredients in a blender and blend until smooth.

2. Serve.

22. Conclusion

Thank you for downloading my book. Hope you enjoyed the recipes! Try It Now! GREEN SMOOTHIES volume 2 coming out soon.

www.ingramcontent.com/pod-product-compliance
Lightning Source LLC
Chambersburg PA
CBHW071300280526
45788CB00004B/1794